First Steps to

ALEXANDER TECHNIQUE

Chris Raff

Tripp Trapp chair courtesy of Backcare Basics @
www.backcarebasics.com

ISBN: 1 86476 101 6

Copyright © Axiom Publishing, 2001.
Unit 2, 1 Union Street, Stepney, South Australia, 5069.

This edition for
SELECT EDITIONS
Devizes
Wiltshire, UK

Alexander Technique Testimonials

When I sing, either in practice or performance, I do at least 20 minutes of Alexander Technique work as part of my warm up. It helps me be aware of what individual parts of my body are doing while I sing.

It also allows my whole body to coordinate and every part participates as it needs to without strain. When it all works everything feels incredibly light and singing becomes much easier than before.
Ben Whittle, 22, Singer.

Sitting eight hours a day in front of a computer terminal over the last ten years, had resulted in back and neck strain. Becoming a pupil of the Alexander Technique, allowed me to become aware of, and improve my body usage at the desk. Within only a few lessons, my back and neck discomfort had eased, and I was no longer prone to the mid-afternoon energy slump.
Robyn Goding, 31, Systems Programmer.

By using the principles of Alexander Technique, I feel flute students learn to play with greater ease and poise. By encouraging an attitude of 'not trying' and improving posture, I believe that most students learn to breathe naturally and develop a more beautiful resonating tonal quality in their flute playing.
Alison Rosser, 55, Advanced Skills Lecturer in Music, Flautist.

The Alexander Technique has improved my body awareness and given me a gentle yet powerful way to improve the way I sit, stand and move. By focusing on thinking, not doing, the technique gets to the heart of the matter. And the 'hands-on' is wonderful!
Benjamin Guerin, 46, Computer Programmer.

Alexander lessons are unique in that they teach the student to recognise and then relax the tightened muscles we all have. These, in turn lead to poor posture.

With the heightened body awareness one is able to constantly work at the relaxation of muscles groups which is necessary for correct use.
M.A. Gould, physiotherapist and Alexander pupil.

Contents
page

Preface

After you have read this book my hope is that you will be inspired to:

Seek more information about the Alexander Technique.

Start exploring some of the ideas and thinking processes I have detailed.

Experiment with the practical (self-help) procedures.

Take lessons from an accredited teacher.

My involvement with the Alexander Technique over the past twenty years has been a rich experience. I continue to rejoice in the pleasure of the free and easy movement it gives. I've been anxious about understanding the essence of the Technique and besotted by the sheer brilliance of its author. Agonised about how best to explain it and amused by its deceptive simplicity. Most of the time intuitively knowing deeply that I have a personal skill of substance that will endure and reward me for the rest of my life.

You may well recognise elements of what I have said as being akin to your own experiences with learning in-depth anything of substance.

For me, this lifelong learning journey continues. For you, I hope your first steps are just the beginning of what is a fascinating and enriching path of recovery and discovery.

Answers to frequently asked questions

What is the Alexander Technique?
This variety of definitions creates a full flavour !

- It's learning to unlearn or undo physical habit patterns that interfere with our natural balance, poise, body alignment and ease of movement.

- A simple, practical process for releasing and redirecting unnecessary tension into useful energy.

- You learn to redirect the use of your body in a thinking way: away from restrictive habits toward freer movement and naturalness.

- The title of Alexander's second book: 'Constructive Conscious Control of the Individual.'

What it is not: The Alexander Technique is not a specific form of exercise, a movement routine or a meditative practice.

Who can benefit from learning the Alexander Technique?
The short answer is 'most people'.

I have worked with children from four years of age to elderly people in their eighties.

Musicians and singers have been traditionally the one occupation to profit from using the Technique. These days, however, more and more people from all walks of life (athletes, office workers, business managers, students, drivers, teachers, parking officers, shearers, artists and craftspeople…) are finding virtue in applying Alexander's principles to themselves in their vocational and recreational activities.

What do people gain from learning the Alexander Technique?

Most people experience a mix of three outcomes:

1. a reduction in the recurrence of specific aches, pains, stresses and strains and consequently more freedom and ease in movement and posture.
2. increasing awareness of the use of the self.
3. improvement in the performance of activities to which they apply the process.

Whether it's the recurring back or neck pain, lack of stamina, inattentiveness, shallow breathing, or interference to the coordination of your golf swing, the Alexander Technique can be gainfully employed to untangle the habits of physical misuse that are quite often the root cause of the problem. Controlling and in many cases eliminating these symptoms can have a significant effect on your outlook.

The Alexander Technique is an educational process. More correctly an ongoing self-educational, psychophysical process, with advantageous spin-offs for performance, consciousness and one's health and well-being.

Who was FM Alexander?

Frederick Matthias Alexander was born in Wynyard Tasmania in 1869. His childhood was spent on a farm in the Table Cape area not far from the town. He was educated in the public school in Wynyard and at 14 he was a school monitor. His father was a blacksmith. In a naturally beautiful environment his life was a happy mix of rural occupations and local 'community'.

In 1885 he moved to Waratah where he had gained employment at the Mt Bischoff tin mine as a junior bookkeeper. His free time was spent participating in local dramatic arts and music productions. In 1888 he was drawn to Melbourne.

Alexander Technique

Melbourne was a prosperous city by this time steeped in the abundance derived from the gold mining industry. The cultural life of the city consequently flourished. While holding down a variety of day jobs, Alexander spent time watching and developing a career in the dramatic arts.

In 1894 he returned to Tasmania touring a recitation program. He went on the road often and as well as giving stage performances, he also offered the local populace tuition in vocal art.

It was also during the 1890's that he started his investigation and private research into the reasons for his recurring bouts of hoarseness. By 1899 Alexander had worked out a process that prevented habits of poor vocal use, such as, sniffing, gasping, pulling the head back and down and breathing shallowly. His discoveries were not confined to just breathing and maintaining good vocal use. His principle extended universally to most human actions: postures, movement and behaviours. Indeed, he had found a technique that could clear away habits of body misuse and restore natural use and poise to the individual. In his case his recurring hoarseness ceased to be a problem and he also reported that his general health improved.

From 1900 to 1904 Alexander resided in Sydney. "Natural elocution" classes and stage work continued until he moved to London.

England was Alexander's home until his death in 1955. He wrote four books in his lifetime and passed on his technique through a training program started in 1930.

He led a full and rich life. He wore many hats: clerk, actor, teacher, tea-taster, punter, horse rider, husband and father.

One of his first assistant teachers, Walter Carrington, remarked that he would say to people who sought his services: 'I think I can be of help to you'. Indeed this self-educational resource – Alexander's technique – has been of assistance to tens of thousands of people throughout the world.

How Does the Alexander Technique Work?

It asks people to become more aware of their body use, determine if that use is detrimental to their stature, coordination or fluidity of movement and, if so, to generate messages to the body to let go, free off and move up. The outcome (of not doing anything physically, like trying to force the body into some 'right' position, but simply communicating with the body,) is to experience subtle physical changes, shifts in balance or weight distribution, or a deeper breath or, sometimes a lighter/taller sense of your self.

It is your conscious registration of these subtle physical changes that is most important. It means your releasing directions, (your way of thinking) have caused a shift or alteration in your experience of yourself. You can feel different because you have undone any number of habits that diminish your poise, natural ease and integration.

To reiterate: the Alexander Technique is a thinking process with physical effects for the better. It's a psychophysical blending. This quality of thinking is what distinguishes it from all other methods, exercise regimes, physical practices and learning modalities.

Another hallmark is that you have a very portable process. You can switch to thinking in an Alexander Technique way in any activity, anywhere, at any time.

Can You Explain More About How It's Applied?

Any occupation can be assisted by the Technique. Habits of misuse are generally unconscious, strong and very sneaky. They definitely need to be pointed out many times so they can be prevented and re-educated. For instance, desk-bound workers slumping in their chair or leaning on their desks is a fairly typical scene. The Alexander Technique teaches them to sit with a condition of balanced uprightness. Similarly with attendants who stand lopsided, they learn how to gently reestablish an even stance. There are people who still bend over with their legs straight and braced. Most are receptive to suggested changes when informed that bending this way, day in and day out, is going to cause recurring back pain, if it has not done so already.

This was one habit of misuse I was made aware of early in my Alexander Technique lessons. It took a while to remember to stop the bad habit of bending from the top of the pelvis and instead direct the head/neck/back upward then bend forward from the hips and counter-balance this lean forward of the torso with appropriate bends in the ankles and knees. With patience and persistence I established this as one of my new ways to bend.

What Does an Alexander Technique Teacher Do?

As an Alexander Technique teacher I explain how people think in a way that can naturally improve how they use their body to perform life's many simple and complex activities.

The Technique doesn't teach people anything new to do. It is not another form of physical exercise. Instead the pupil is taught how to be more kinaesthetically aware of what they are doing. Once pointed out, habits of body misuse become apparent. Some examples being uneven stances, jutting out of the lower jaw, one shoulder higher than the other, various strains in the back or legs and tightness in the neck.

The pupil comes to appreciate that these habits are interference to the poise of the head and the lengthening of the spine (Alexander's principle of the primary control). The use of thought to prevent these misuses while also promoting consciously an integrating direction for the head-neck-back relationship to move toward, gives the pupil an experience of subtle change in their physical condition. Various responses are reported: "I feel less heavy", "my breathing is fuller", "I am taller", "that back pain I mentioned has reduced", "I feel more together".

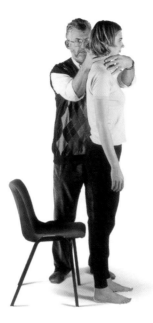

Gentle guidance through the use of the teacher's hands coupled with verbal cues conveys this thinking process. It is repeated again and again in different activities throughout the lesson. The pupil is expected to apply this process often away from their lessons. Gradually, by learning to stop and think, habits that cause recurring aches and pains or that diminish the quality of performance in sports, music, vocational and everyday activities are re-educated.

The Alexander Technique becomes a constructive way to choose to think. This skill alerts us to our misuses and gives us the option to change our condition. As well we can use it to effortlessly maintain a high degree of poise in our bearing and carriage. For the pupil increasingly more natural body use positively affects the way they function in daily activities.

Alexander's Discoveries

If not for his sheer brilliance then for his dogged determination, it is important to acknowledge and pay tribute to Alexander's pioneering work. He was a genius. This should become more apparent once you have read this interpretation of how he blends his observations, ideas, concepts and principles into what is called the Alexander Technique.

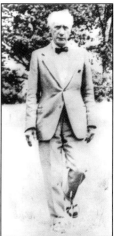

Essentially he has given us a technique that can allow our body, our sense of ourselves, to move toward a condition of poise, ease, alignment and integration without force or effort. This is accomplished by using the conscious process of thinking he developed which can override the way we automatically act and react to life's stimuli.

Whether it is to read more about the Technique or to start applying it, the following should be helpful amplification of his work. If you wish to read the master himself, I would suggest you start with his book *The Use of the Self*. Chapter 1 is titled 'Evolution of a Technique' and is a retrospective account of his discovery process.

As with anything original, a particular language emerges. Alexander drew on his experiences with stage work and horses to express his findings.

Primary Control

You will strike this concept often in the work. It is a fundamental.

Basically it coordinates the whole body.

It is the dynamic relationship between your head and neck, and that relationship to the rest of the body.
Alexander stated his principle this way:
'…the true and primary movement in each and every act.'

How does this dynamic work?

Our head weighs between 4 and 6 kilograms. It sits on the top of the spine at the atlanto-occipital joint. The skull pivots at this point.

The centre of gravity of your skull is up and forward of the alanto-occipital joint. You have 2/3rds of the weight of the skull in front of the pivot point.

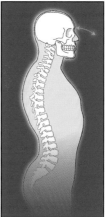

It explains why when we go to sleep sitting up our head generally drops onto our chest.

When we are awake our head perches on the top of the spine and if we are not looking at anything in particular then our view is roughly straight ahead. This is maintained by a constant interplay within our neck muscles. It's falling forward, out of balance, being corrected only to lose balance again, to be corrected again…

This minuscule movement happens regardless of whether the head is turned or not. It's a very fine tuning. We don't register this movement consciously.

The quality of the work being done by the neck muscles is really important. It determines how the head balances. It can be free or quite tight.

We interfere with this quality in many ways. The underlying villain is our forceful habits of misuse. If I have a habit of jutting my chin out and tightening muscles in the back of my neck, then I am restricting the muscles that help maintain the dynamic balance of the head on top of the spine. This habit may be apparent when I am sitting, speaking or moving.

In my case the profile view of my head/neck relationship depicted a neck angled out and forward from my torso at about 20°. From the frontal view the neck inclined right and the head tilted back to the left to make me level headed.

I believe this misshapen appearance developed slowly in my primary and secondary school years. My sitting posture was never corrected from leaning on the desk in a collapsed twist (right shoulder coming around and down as I held my pen, my right foot crossed my left ankle). Writing in this position became normal. Any other position

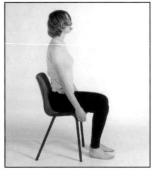

was uncomfortable. Add to this habit another, that of looking up to copy from the blackboard without changing the overall posture. This meant lifting and turning my head up and to the right, seeing what had to be copied and then dropping the head down into my twisted frame again, and again and again...

When I demonstrate the dynamic head-neck-back relationship to pupils in front of a mirror they are astonished at how they have distorted the way the head sits on the top of the spine. The insidious creep of habits into what we do makes us unconscious of them hence the slight shock when the neck muscles are coaxed to release (via the teacher's touch and verbal cues) and the head is able to regain freer balance. This subtle change triggers other changes, shifts or alterations in the body. Of course it varies from person to person.

The way to get this release happening is not by doing anything physical like pulling the chin in or holding the head erect. The undoing of the imbalances and displacement of the head-neck-back relationship is achieved by mental cues, and non-manipulative directions from a teacher's hands.

Away from lessons you are expected to explore and experiment with giving directions to yourself without forcing or making any effort. More about this later. Gradually, with patience and persistence, you regain a more poised head. As the main frame of yourself restores its togetherness, other parts (be it limbs, jaw, pelvis shoulder girdle, or the respiratory system) fall back into a more natural placement. Rounded shoulders, shallow breathing, or tense legs, for instance, can be gently altered for the better.

As Alexander said: "We can throw away the habit of a lifetime in a few minutes if we use our brains." What he didn't say was that you have to provoke this use of your brain again and again!

Use Affects Functioning

When hearing people describe other people you may hear comments like, 'hanging about', 'down in the dumps', 'got the slouches', 'she moves with such elegance', 'he has a dignified appearance', 'the rowers moved as one; with a graceful style and poise'.

Use refers to the posture or the coordination and movement of animals and humans. As well, our behaviours are a component of our use. In particular our reactive behaviours, to such things as, dropping something on the ground, rising from a chair, or hear our name mentioned, or, when, in the middle of the night, we think we hear an intruder, or what the thought of giving that speech or musical performance transmits to our body.

To quote Alexander: 'Talk about a man's individuality and character: it's the way he uses himself'. There is no real separation of the self into exclusively physical or mental components. We are, as Alexander calls it, psychophysical entities and use ourselves as such.

Functioning is how we perform or operate part of, or the whole of, our self in any activity. This can be how we breathe when at rest to how we move when riding a bicycle very fast.

Poor use, and misuse, is approaching epidemic proportions.

If I slump, my use (the slump) affects or influences my functioning. One element of this posture is the rounded shoulders/collapsed chest, diminishing and restricting my breathing.

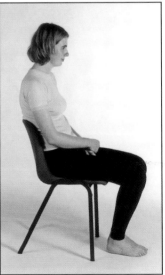

If, every time I drop something, I react instantly by bending over (with my legs held straight) then my use, or more correctly, my misuse, will affect my functioning. Maybe not at that time but in this case the habit will eventually cause my lower back to complain.

Good use is a rare sight. Indeed I have been asked when sitting in a balanced and easy uprightness if something was wrong with my back. We lack role models for good use. Manual handling has to be taught as an occupational health and safety requirement because people have no basic rules or principles upon which to rely, let alone apply, when lifting, transferring, holding or pushing.

Our eye can catch the exquisite walker moving in a smooth glide before us. Toddlers are exemplary; most bend and carry themselves with enviable deportment. Our attraction to observing topnotch athletes and performing artists is in part due to their ability to make what they do look poised, easy and naturally efficient. Referring back to the dynamic head-neck-back relationship, when good use is apparent, the whole muscular system is operating as a complete unit.

For most people, in varying degrees, our use is interfering with our functioning. We have acquired habits of misuse that we are either ignorant of or at best, only partially aware of.

Alexander falls into this latter case. His repeated loss of voice caused him to eventually ask his doctor: "Is it not fair, then to conclude that it was something I was doing that evening in using my voice that was the cause of the trouble?"

Like many people, including myself who undertake Alexander lessons, we have decided to investigate the possibility that the recurrence of the problem is due to our use. By this stage we know the symptoms can be temporarily appeased by various treatments but what we are now seeking is a remedy for the cause.

If our formative education had dealt with the principles of movement and a conscious and repeated development of our kinaesthetic sense, then we would be better placed to be aware of our misuses and how to prevent them.

Unfortunately this is not the case even today. Physical educators steer their students in the direction of exercise and sports skill acquisition. Some worthwhile work, though under-funded, is being done to effectively remedy children who are poorly coordinated.

This problem will continue until educators realise that F. M. Alexander discovered a number of principles about human movement and behaviour that are well worth promoting and need to be passed on to our young people as part of their personal skills repertoire.

Here are some axioms for good use that have emerged from studying and applying the Alexander Technique.

"The head leads and the body follows."
"When sitting, sit in balance on your sitting bones."
"The periphery of the limb (fingers and toes) lead the limb into movement."
"When sitting it is best to have the knees lower than the hip joints."
"The senses of sight, sound, smell and taste lead the head to lead the body into movement."

In addition to knowing how we are structured and how we are designed to function, being more attuned kinaesthetically is extremely valuable to the individual.

If you can appreciate poise, balance, fluidity in movement, ease and a sense of physical integrity, then you will know when a condition less than this visits you.

Again knowing and applying the Alexander Technique can advise you what stimulus, what action, what reaction causes you to fall from poise and ease and, if you so choose, how to deal with this unsatisfactory experience.

Sensory Appreciation

We apprehend and experience our world through our senses. Traditionally we are taught there are five senses. We know there are more. 'A sense of belonging', or 'intuitively I sensed something amiss', or 'I felt myself lose balance', are other senses.

The latter is part of what some call the sixth sense, the kinesthetic sense. That is the sense of position and movement of parts of our self or our whole self. This 'muscle sense' informs us and gives us a feel for balance, position, motion, resistance, weight bearing…it gives us an inner picture of our use.

The kinesthetic sense is somewhat downtrodden in our culture. We use it well in our preschool years but it becomes overridden by visual and auditory inputs as we get older. It doesn't get the attention it deserves. We don't have an in-built daily dance like other cultures. If more inner-directed movement routines like tai chi or yoga were part of our physical culture then the kinesthetic sense would be more prominent in our awareness.

This is not the case, and part of learning the Alexander Technique requires a development of attention to this sense. A strong awareness of how we are balanced or not, the degree of appropriate or inappropriate tension present for a particular activity and awareness of flowing or gauche coordination are all parts of a growing kinesthetic sense of ourselves.

When reading Alexander or other sources the phrases 'unreliable sensory appreciation', 'faulty sensory appreciation' or 'debauched kinaesthia' will recur a lot.

Many people are aware how they sense themselves is not how they appear. Photos to some extent, but definitely video playback of ourselves, make most of us self-conscious and sometimes a little shocked at the way we move or posture ourselves. Equally the caught glimpse of our self in the departmental store window as we walk past can require a second check to make sure it is who we think it is!

What's being discussed is unreliable sensory appreciation. Alexander coined this as a way of describing how the kinesthetic sense goes awry. During his period of observation in the 1890's he used a three-way mirror system to watch himself in profile. It meant he didn't have to turn his head to see his movement pattern in profile. What astonished him from the outset was the amount of movement he made when he projected his voice. He thought he only pulled his head back slightly, the mirror told him it was much larger movement than he thought. Hence the quote: 'sensory appreciation conditions conception – you can't know a thing by an instrument that is wrong.'

At a refined level our kinesthetic sense lies to us about our position and movements. Here is a dilemma. What do we rely upon to gauge if we are sitting correctly or moving with restriction? Our habitual use suggests all is well, but mirrors, video feedback or a coach/teacher tells us that it simply isn't the way we think it is. So how do we know we are getting back to a better use of ourselves?

Heightening our appreciation of our kinesthetic sense is still important despite its faulty nature. So attuned we can quickly register change, difference, shift or alteration in our state of balance, alignment, quality of movement or integration achieved by thinking in the way Alexander suggests.

'There is no such thing as a right position, but there is such a thing as a right direction.' In other words Alexander is saying this: "If I think in such a way that I sense (register) myself moving away from my habit of misuse toward a condition that's not familiar, or either more or less comfortable, and certainly not 'normal', but perhaps more natural, then I am on my way toward good use of myself. I am heading in the 'right direction.'"

Trying to make myself feel right is not going to help me reeducate my habits of misuse. Feeling for it (the correct posture or way of moving) needs to be checked and replaced by reasoning out what needs to occur and then I consciously guide myself in that direction. An instinctive reaction is replaced by reasoned response. This may seen a long way around to solve a problem but it's the best one I know of to make lasting change.

The way of thinking developed by Alexander also involves understanding the terms: inhibition, direction and means whereby.

Inhibition
We can change nothing if we don't stop doing what we habitually do.

Alexander says: 'you can't do something you don't know, if you keep on doing what you do know.'

To get into new territory, to make new inner programming possible, to prevent the old from recurring, we have to withhold consent to do what we automatically or instinctively do.

For example, if I drop my pen on the floor my impulse is to pick it up straight away. This is a well-established stimulus-response pattern. I swoop down to retrieve the pen. Prior to Alexander lessons I would have thought nothing of this activity. Post Alexander lessons I examine what my instinctive reaction does to me. My body awareness tells me as I do this movement I am rounding my back, I am straining to maintain balance, I am twisting my torso and I feel weighted down. If instead I inhibit this reaction I have an infinite number of choices about how I will pick up the dropped pen.

Application of this inhibition principle is far reaching. We can't completely manage circumstances, situations, other people's actions and events in our daily round. However we can manage our responses to them. Our reaction to the phone ringing may be to rush to pick it up. If you inhibit that reaction you could choose to calmly walk to where the phone is and answer it. You could decide to wait until the sixth ring before answering it or you could decide to let it ring out. By inhibiting you have created the possibility of new responses to the stimulus. In other words you have chosen to respond rather than react to the situation.

By spending a little time analysing your pattern of reaction to a selection of stimuli during your day, you can find some that impinge upon your good use. Alexander puts it this way: 'you translate everything, whether physical or mental or spiritual into muscular tension.' So the way you habitually react to a stimulus can be assessed kinaesthetically and determined beneficial (no appreciable tightening or strain) or detrimental (yes, I detect pulling down and tension in the neck and shoulders). If the latter then some reeducation on your part may be a good choice.

Essentially, inhibition as prescribed by Alexander, gives us the chance, the time and space, to choose our responses to any stimulus. A choice he suggests is to bring conscious direction to our actions in order to maintain good use and reeducate poor use.

Direction/s

Thinking about where you want your body to go, what you want your body to do and not do, and how you want it to be gives a general overview of this notion.

'Giving directions' is a mental process Alexander developed to offset or prevent his habits of misuse and encourage or promote good use of the whole self. These directions trigger a change in the body. Generally it is a subtle change hence the need to be kinaesthetically aware. For instance, the outcome of giving directions may be that your breathing is slightly deeper, your weight bearing may shift or your shoulder might drop. On some occasions the experience is profound. The body seemingly draws itself together so much so that you strongly sense yourself more integrated, aligned and poised.

It was via this process that Alexander was able to recite without falling into his habitual pattern of pulling his head back and down, depressing his larynx, gasping for breath, lifting his chest and tightening his legs.

How do you give directions? Inwardly saying, picturing or sensing (or a combination of these faculties), 'neck free, head to go forward and up, back to lengthen and widening' is a good start.

Remember it's a mental process, there is no physical effort or doing involved. This is difficult to understand and trust initially but as your awareness develops and you allow the releases to occur, wherever the body decides, you can find yourself moving into a different experience of your self.

Here's a practical process I do that amplifies what I am saying.

When driving to the city I sometimes choose to use the wait at a red light to do some Alexander work on myself. First I assume that I am misusing myself as I am sitting behind the steering wheel.

I inhibit any desire to immediately change my position, then I observe myself kinaesthetically. What do I notice about tension in my jaw/chin area? Are my shoulders relaxed? How am I sitting? Are my hands over tense?

Alexander Technique

Next I give my directions: 'Neck free, head to go up and forward, jaw release, shoulders widen, legs ease…,' I recall experiences of letting go of tension in some parts of my body, I use pictures of the head delicately balancing on the top of the spine, I ask the shoulders to be broad… Almost without exception I sense the jaw let go of some tension, next there is a very slight drop of holding in the shoulders and sometimes I feel the hands soften to a less tense grasp of the wheel. These releases are directed into the head moving up and the whole body following, this in turn at least reminds me of my overall direction and at most restores a strong sense of poise.

I might choose to think like this six or seven times during the hour-long journey. This is just one application of the Technique amongst many that I instigate throughout my day. The cumulative effect of thinking like this is less unnecessary stress and strain and more association with poise and freedom in the body.

Alexander opens up a new dimension to our movement. It is best expressed in the question: Where am I heading and how am I going to use myself as I go there?

Endgaining and the Means Whereby
'Goal oriented', 'outcome focused', or 'just do it' are modern ways of expressing endgaining as Alexander saw it in his day.

It's rushing to our end and not considering the process – the means whereby – for getting there. Of course acting quickly in emergency situations or spontaneously in social settings has its place.

What Alexander wants people to appreciate is that due consideration to the process, that is, enjoying the journey and not dwelling on arriving, has profound effects on our use of ourselves.

For a start it makes us more present and conscious of our actions

Let's say your end to gain (goal) is to reach out for a book on a high shelf. If you were observing yourself just doing it, it is quite likely you would find yourself compromising the head-neck-back relationship. This could be a dropping of the head over to one side, lifting your shoulders and twisting your torso. You could well have discovered a prevalent habit of misuse. Anyway you get what you need – the book – but at what expense to your physical integrity?

If instead you were to stop (inhibit) your immediate impulse to reach for the book and consider how you'd manage to get it (the means whereby) you'd possibly sequence your actions. You may even realise that you need to get closer to the shelf as better place to start the reach. You give your directions to maintain the dynamic head-neck-back relationship. You let the hand lead the arm to reach up for the book. If it's still out of reach you don't strain or swivel your body, but go onto your tip-toes, still maintaining balance and a front-on frame to the bookshelf. If it's still out of reach, get a step or chair to stand on!

This may seem overly tedious. If you want to change habits of use for the better then some dedicated work is necessary in the early stages of applying the Alexander Technique. Many old bad habits of use evaporate as you 'think in activity'. As you realise you are going to have to reach up for something, you recall the means whereby previously established and reapply them in the current situation. You build a portfolio for good use in daily activities.

This tour of Alexander's discoveries, observations and principles is not comprehensive. It can assist in getting you started in practical ways and pave the way for further investigation into this unique technique.

What Can I do For Myself

Let's look at this next step in four ways:

- Observation
- Inlook/Outlook
- Body mapping 1. Vitalising the kinesthetic sense.
              2. Anatomy.
- Procedures   1. Constructively resting the back.
              2. Out of slumped sitting.

If you've got this far in the book then my assumption is that you are, or would be, prepared to take more responsibility for your health, well being and self development.

Taking this responsibility is also taking more control of your life. It's what Alexander decided and it's what I've done (and continue to do), that is, question the use of myself.

What is it that I am doing in the use of myself that could be causing (any number of these):
- Recurring aches and pains in various parts of my body?
- Accumulating stress and strains?
- A lack of fluidity or naturalness in performance?
- The repetition of a behaviour pattern?

What can I do about these patterns/habits?

Observation
Self observations
Get acquainted. Get to know your habits and patterns of use. Observe yourself as you are.

If it's a recurring pain in the neck, start noticing your sleep positions. Do I lie on one side more than the other? Does the top arm, when sleeping on my side, drape and pull my shoulder and neck muscles? Is my pillow too high or too low?

Question: how do I move when getting out of different sorts of chairs? If a swivel chair, do I turn to the right most of the time? Is this a preference or is it the way my workstation is set up? What leads the turn: my pelvis or my chest or my chin or my eyes?

Often you do discover patterns. Could they be the underlying cause of your symptom, the pain in the neck? You might even figure out how a particular habit negatively affects your wholeness, the dynamic relationship between your head and neck and that relationship to your back. Alexander said that if we can "prevent the things we have been doing then we are halfway home".

Other observations

Another form of observation is consciously choosing to observe others. How's this helpful? Human beings have developed some incredibly interesting variations on the themes of walking, bending or standing.

Non-critically watch the passing parade from a park seat or a bench in a shopping mall. Ask yourself, "what would I have to do to move like that person? How would I feel if I moved like that? How do I do that movement anyway?"

Visual observations.

Visual aids are also useful for putting your attention on your posture and actions. Alexander cleverly used a three-way mirror system so he could see himself in profile without having to turn his head.

You could do the same, but these days many people have access to video cameras and once you've got over trying to move how you think you should for the camera, you can gain interesting feedback about your 'normal' body use.

Alexander Technique

In group teaching of the Alexander Technique, I do a 3 to 4 minutes walking observation activity in which one person walks about three paces ahead of a course colleague. The follower imitates the person's walk then shows the leader how they see their walking style. The process causes lots of laughter but does give the leader interesting feedback and insights. In many cases participants report a new awareness of habits associated with their walking style.

Do ask other people to give you input on how they observe you. I encourage business teams to agree to interchange impressions of how their colleagues are sitting. "I feel upright, do I look upright?". Remember it is very likely what you feel you are doing is not quite the way it is actually.

Inlook/Outlook
- An open mind.
- Self acceptance.
- Non-judgmental awareness.
- A willingness to explore and experiment with new or different ideas and activities.
- Flexible thinking.

If you consider you are moving toward these mental states, then learning the Alexander Technique will be on your wavelength.

In retrospect my mental states were hardly in tune with those stated above. Indeed I was a challenge to my teachers. I constantly tried to get it right. I was very self-critical when it didn't work as I thought it 'should' have. Truly the antithesis of Alexander's teaching. So I do believe the Alexander Technique has made these states more available to me. Also, I realise that these states are relative for everyone. Implicitly they need constant review and renewal otherwise I would not continue to learn and teach the Technique.

Any activities that cultivate a movement toward these mental states are encouraged. Edward De Bono's lateral thinking exercises, the "Inner Game of …" books, various meditations, martial arts, doing something unusual for yourself like learning to juggle are some examples that develop components of the attitudes suggested.

Body Mapping
Important too is the appreciation of your kinesthetic sense. This is mentioned in chapter 3 under Alexander's discoveries. It's your muscle sense or movement sense. It tells you where you are in space, how you're moving or if stationary how your posture feels.

Many people taking up tai chi or yoga for the first time in their later years of life get tremendous pleasure from these disciplines as they generate suppleness and vitality. Many sense themselves being reunited with a lost part of themselves, that is, their kinesthetic sense. It is in your interest to cultivate more awareness of this sense.

Let's use an example to explain why.

You are standing in a bank queue. Nothing to do but wait! Why not apply some Alexander thinking to the activity. The start point is to observe kinaestheticly. That is, you tune into your experience of weight bearing (is one leg taking most of my weight?), don't change your position just yet, what else can I notice (do I feel strain in the lower back? Is there a twist in my torso? Am I light, heavy or in between?)

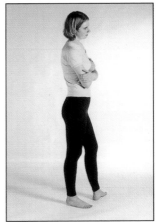

All the questions are highlighting your kinesthetic sense. With time and practice you become adept at detecting unnecessary tension in your body. You can then think in a way to undo the interference, in the case of our example, to easy, balanced standing. After your observations you then give directions and allow the body to move to restore more even uprightness in your stance.

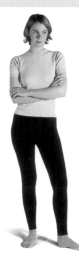

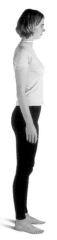

Training your attention to be kinaestheticly aware is a continual process. It's like an auto-pilot.

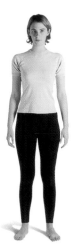

As you move away from poise the kinesthetic alarm rings, you correct (by giving directions), moving back toward poise for a time, then your kinesthetic attention is deflected, then off goes the alarm again, and again you have the choice to correct. As you gain more kinesthetic appreciation, the consequence is that the distance between going off course (the increased tensions we make when we are not balanced for instance) and making the correction, becomes less and less.

Body pictures.
Your inner maps of yourself may need some correction and enrichment.

Are the bits of you where you think they are? At some point in teaching I ask people to show me where they think their hip joints are. In most cases they point to the topside of their pelvis. This is a good 12cm above the hip joint. Ask that person to bend at the hips and they bend in the lower back. Using the hips as a hinge to bend from is a better option.

The point is that many of us don't have a basic appreciation of our anatomy and physiology. Knowing something of our design, structure and function is very helpful in learning the Alexander Technique.

Lessons
The process of learning the Alexander Technique is shortened if you decide to take a course of lessons. How many depends on what outcomes you want. Some people have seven or eight and stop because that's enough to learn how to prevent the recurring neck or back pain. Others take the recommended course of 20 to 30 lessons. After this some keep coming weekly or fortnightly or monthly or half-yearly either because lessons are a part of their health maintenance plan or they wish to refine, refresh and/or review the skill they have learnt.

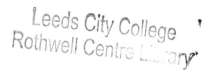

Two Self-Help Procedures

1. The semi-supine position
The position of maximum rest for the back.

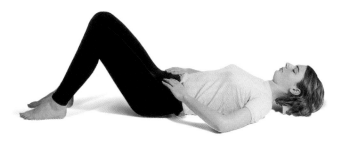

The semi-supine position can have positive outcomes for our health and well being if done daily. It can do any or all of the following:

Rest the back
The surface you lie on needs to be firm. A yoga mat or a carpeted floor is ideal. A bed is not good as it is not firm and does not make the body respond to its surface.

Restore length to the spine
When we are in upright positions during the day the downward pressure of gravity and other factors tend to shorten the spine. Fluid that resides in the intervertebral disks is squeezed out during the day and is absorbed by the vertebra below the disk. Lying on a firm surface in semi-supine allows some of this fluid to drain back into the disks quite quickly. This does not restore the disks to the fullness that comes from a good nights sleep. It does arrest the draining of fluid and restores some for the fluid to the disks. The speed with which the fluid drains back is initially fast. This reduces with time so after 30 minutes in the position the drainage has slowed to almost nothing. I consider 20 to 25 minutes to be the optimal amount of time in the position.

Opens the rib cage

The firmness of the surface you lie on causes the rib cage to widen and as a consequence can deepen our breathing.

Re-align the body

With regular practice the position can rebalance the body. It is as if the ground and gravity conspire to gently untangle your twists and unevenness.

Release unnecessary tension

By being still in the position patterns of tension are revealed. People are surprised about how much tension they unconsciously hold in their body. Gritted teeth, scrunched toes, gripped hands, shoulders braced, tight buttocks…are some discoveries people make.

Induce physical stillness

Initially it is usual to find this position a bit hard on the body. It doesn't take it long to accommodate this. As well, some people are fidgety. This too passes. After a few weeks of regular semi-supines, most people find the body enjoys the position.

Quieten the mind

While you are in semi-supine you can mentally direct your attention to your weight bearing points or your muscles in the head/neck region or to your joints. This not only enhances body awareness it also has the effect of single tracking the mind. A little similar to meditation in that it makes the present moment the main focus and shuts down a lot of mental chatter on past and future matters. The outcome can be quite therapeutic.

Most people who regularly practice semi-supine swear by its value. Given what's been advanced above it's well worth a trial. Please remember it's to be enjoyed not endured. If you feel sore after doing it for twenty minutes the first time, cut the time back to 10 minutes for a few times and see if that is all right. If so gradually increase the time to 20 minutes.

Alexander Technique

You may wonder why getting down into and up from the floor is such a 'by numbers' routine. Here are some reasons:

1. It stops you rushing and possibly hurting yourself.
2. It makes you think in a sequential way.
3. The whole process reinforces many of Alexander's ideas in practice.

The assumption is that you don't have sore knees or wrists.

You will need:

        A quiet, draft-free space
        At least 20 minutes
        A firm, flat surface
        3 or 4 paperback books (4-5cm thick)
        to be warmly dressed

To know how many books you need under your head, do the following. Stand with you back to a firm wall. The heels of your feet about 3cm from the skirting board. Fall back onto the wall and get a friend to measure the distance from the back of your head to the wall. This should give a good approximation of the thickness of books you need.

It may help you to make a recording of the following steps and play them through until it becomes second nature.

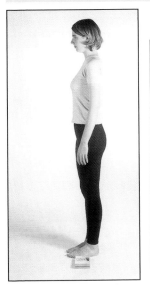

1. Place the books on the floor and stand beside them.

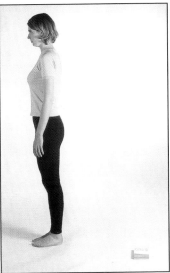

2. Think up through your body and take 2 large steps forward.

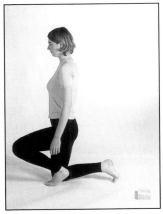

3. Pause, think up before kneeling on one knee and then the other knee,

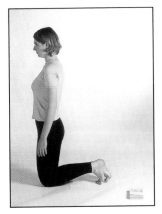

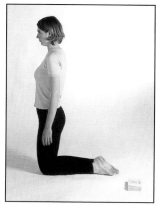

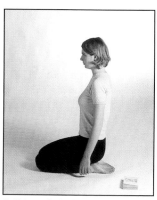

4. Let the toes release their pivot so the top of the toes are contacting the floor.

5. Release in the hip joints and sit on you heels.
Gently let the eyes lead the head to the side you think the books are on, sight the books.

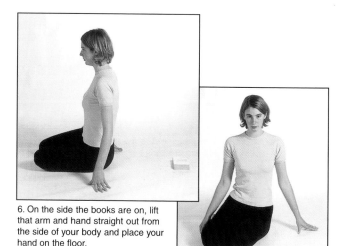

6. On the side the books are on, lift that arm and hand straight out from the side of your body and place your hand on the floor.

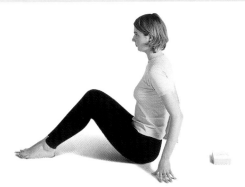

7. Use this hand and arm to support yourself as you slide your buttocks off your heels and sit on your bottom.

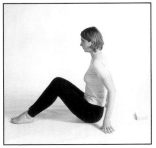

8. Keeping the legs bent swing them around and in front of you.
 Place the other arm and hand straight out from your side and use it to support you.
Gently let the eyes lead the head to sight the books again.
Using both hands and arms, lift yourself to where you think you need to be to land with your head on the books when you roll out. (it is better to do this than grope around for the books as that action will strain your neck/shoulder region).

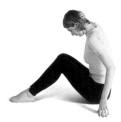

9. Drop your head onto your chest and lean your torso forward. (this removes a degree of strain in the upper body)
Place a hand behind your head (this is to support your head and stop neck strain as you roll out and down onto the books).

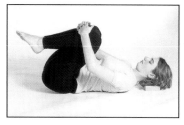

10. In your mind picture your spine rolling out and down onto the floor. Then actually roll out onto the floor.
Use your other hand/arm to locate the books and place them under the back of the skull.

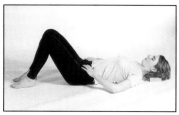

11. Let the head rest comfortably on the books, wriggle the shoulders to get them comfortable and then feel with flat hands for the degree of hollow in the lower back region. You shouldn't lift any part of yourself to do this.
If you have a hollow in the lower back region then gently raise your knees toward your chest so you can hug them. This action should shift the pelvis slightly (a pelvic tilt) to gain a flatter back. If you don't feel you've got more back on the ground after doing this, please don't force the pelvis to stay tilted or try to push the back into the floor. Be patient and in time a flatter lower back should occur as you get used to the position. Please remember semi-supine is a position of maximum rest for the back or a balanced resting position, any forcing or pushing is contrary to that outcome.

12. After hugging your knees, place the feet flat on the floor close to your buttocks. Do this in such a way so that the knees will not fall outward.
Rest you hands on your pelvis. Make any final adjustment to the height of the books. Then let yourself be still. You should not be making any effort anywhere.
Observe, inwardly tour, your weight bearing points, muscles in the head/neck region and your joints for the next 20 minutes.

Getting out of semi-supine

Before you start, think through what follows first, and then proceed.

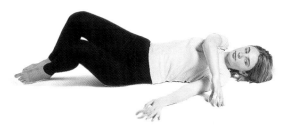

1. Let the eyes lead the head to side you are rolling to. (Avoid lifting you head up off the books prematurely as this can cause strain in the neck.)
As your head is rolling, lift the appropriate arm across the body and allow its momentum to continue your spiral roll. At some point you will need to make a little effort to get yourself into the all fours position.

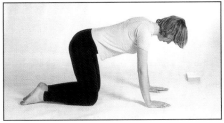

2. Pause here and check the following: are my knees under my hips? Are my hands under my face? Is my face parallel to the ground? Is my neck lifted? Is my lower back flat? If not adjust gently.

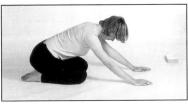
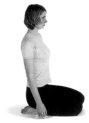

3. Rock back onto your heels

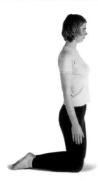

4. Stand on your knees

5. Tuck the toes forward to pivot them

6. Bring one knee up

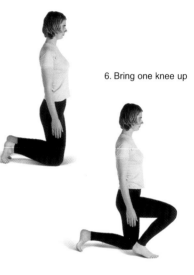

7. Lift yourself into standing by either going forward and up or back and up.
Take a short walk to get the body moving again. Also take a moment to appreciate the outcomes of your twenty minutes in semi-supine.

An aside note here, the eyes leading the head to roll over and out of semi-supine can be carried over into your turning from side to side in bed and getting out of bed. It's simply following the principle 'the head leads and the body follows'. My youthful habit was to throw the legs out of bed first and let the torso catch up. For principled reasons I no longer get out of bed this way.

2. Getting out of a slump

The habit of slumping or slouching in sitting is an epidemic. Of course, officially, this has not been acknowledged by the health authorities. Anyone who stops and looks at any audience, classroom of children or congregation will see few people sitting in an upright and balanced state.

Slumping down and then thrusting the torso up to correct the slump is a dilemma for most of us. Slumping is known to be bad and sitting up straight is strenuous and difficult to maintain. Slumping is the other and, ah yes, relieving option.

A word here about chairs. Take heed. The chairs provided may be a health hazard. They are if they have seats that slant downwards toward the back and the actual back of the chair is far from being perpendicular. If you are doing this procedure on one of these chairs, generally plastic moulded chairs, then the value of this procedure is reduced. The reason is that the chair is encouraging you to slouch by its design. Consequently your re-educational efforts to stop slumping are short-circuited by the chair.

Back to the procedure. We get into a habitual loop, 'sitting up straight' and slumping down. Again and again this happens. It's worth investigating if the part of your body you use to lift yourself into sitting up straight is possibly a point where you get recurring pain. If this is the case, as it is for many people, then this procedure can prevent this habit of misuse as well.

To break this loopy habit you need a new option.

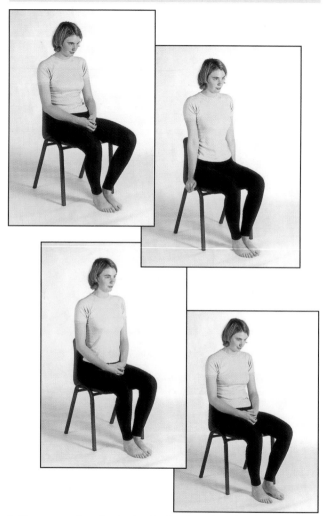

1. Stop your usual reaction to slumping (most people push or thrust themselves into sitting upright) and instead look down with your eyes before dropping your head onto your chest.

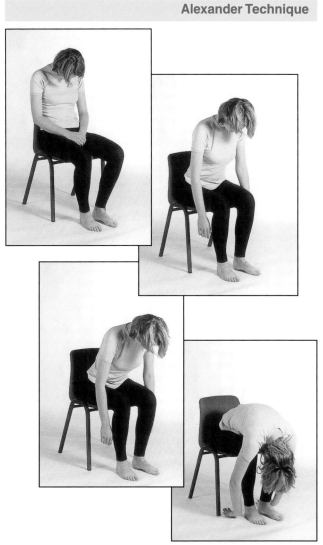

2. Slowly lean forward from the hips (as far as is practical). In ideal surroundings you would be able to drop your head between your knees.

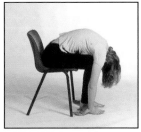

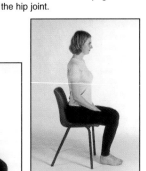

3. Allow the weight of the dropped head to lead your torso forward, out and down. so that, even though your back is curved, you sense the weight of the head lengthening the spine.
If possible let your arms dangle at your sides.
Remember there is no forcing. Just unravelling, releasing muscles.
Continue to think this as you...

4. Ease back into the upright from the hip joint.

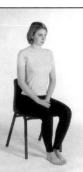

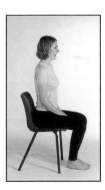

5. To sit easily with an aligned head-neck-back profile.
Keep in mind the thought of the head and torso moving upward.
Test your balance in sitting by slightly rocking on your sitting bones.
Release any acquired tension in the jaw, shoulders and the back of the pelvis.

Congratulations! You have negotiated a procedure that will eventually become second nature and less dramatic. It is set out above in ideal surroundings but with a little creative thought you can modify it for theatre seats, cafes, cars and at your desk.

Hints and Tips

Children and parents
I offer parents of children under about the age of 13 the following suggestions.

Strollers/Pushers
As a L Plate parent I was to learn the hard way regarding these pieces of apparatus. The one we got looked good and ran well in the store. After a few weeks my wrists complained of strain. This particular stroller didn't have proper handles but rather a padded handle bar. This meant a lot of force through the hands and arms was needed to negotiate kerbs, bumps and grass. The wheels didn't always go where you wanted them to so this added to the difficulty. Contemporary strollers/pushers are more stable and manoeuvrable. I would ask to road test it outside the store just to be sure it rides well and you can manipulate it with ease.

Reaching
Most houses are designed with big people in mind. This makes life difficult for little people. We can do a few small things to make them more even in the use of their body around the home. Small stools they can stand on at the bathroom basin or in the kitchen at the sink or bench can avert overreaching and twisting the torso unduly. Footrests (a small stool, a bar on the chair or 'phone books) when sitting at a table or at a desk can help maintain uprightness.

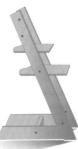

The Tripp-Trapp chair is a great addition to young families. It can double as a highchair or a stool as the child gets older.

Touch Typing

Who knows how long the keyboard is going to be around. Regardless of the developments in word processing via voice activation, I would recommend your offspring learn to touch type. Hunting and pecking the keys is a disaster. Looking down and up all the time really takes a toll on the neck muscles.

Backpacks

They need to be worn as they are designed; two straps over two shoulders.

There comes a point when children are just carrying too much weight in their backpack. Keep an eye on this as it varies for each child. If they appear loaded down they probably are. A heavy backpack coupled with slinging it over one shoulder every day and you have a recipe for curvature of the spine.

A great innovation in baggage is the small bag/case that you can wheel. A retractable arm is pulled out and the case is pulled along on small built-in wheels. It can be easily picked up by a handle when necessary. It's a must for the frequent traveller. It could also be a solution for school children who have to cart books and sports equipment to and from school everyday.

Breathing

Alexander did not tell us how to breathe. He did observe the misuses that can interfere with our natural breathing mechanism. The habit of sniffing strongly or gasping to take in breath is not helpful to our state of ease in the head/neck region.

Unless we are really short of breath, the shoulders should not be moving up and down excessively when we breathe.

It is preferable to breathe in through the nose, this way the air is being filtered, warmed and moistened assuming it's cold dry air we are breathing. The breath fills the lungs which in turn pushes the diaphragm down, This dome-like muscle, positioned up and under the rib cage, expands the lower rib cage so you see movement in the midriff area: not a lot in the front of the torso but more on the sides and in the mid/lower back.

If you observe your child mouth breathing it's for the best to ask him or her to shut the lips and let the air come in through the nose. Exhalation is either through the mouth or the nose.

Desks and chairs

Think ergonomic when buying desks and chairs for the family.

Ideally when sitting at a desk we are in an upright balanced posture, our elbows are slightly higher than the desktop or the keyboard and our feet are flat on the floor.

For chairs, height and angles for seat and back need to be adjustable. It caters for comfort. It also allows for growth. Adjustable height desks are not easy to find. You can put blocks of wood under the legs to increase the height, but short of sawing pieces off the legs, lowering the height is difficult. It means we change the height of the chair to attain the desired configuration. For short people this generally means the feet need to be on a footrest or telephone books. If the feet are not placed evenly on the floor the support for the legs has to come from somewhere else. That's right, the back is taxed.

The posture we do our work from is the position attained from the "out of a Slump process" discussed earlier. It is worth insisting this be the best way to work. As a parent the odds are stacked against you though. Can you practice what you preach about sitting up? Children are great imitators and adopt the immediate and prevailing postures and movement patterns of their parents.

Thankfully school chairs are changing for the better; flat seats and fairly upright backs. The plastic moulded chairs that have a dipped seat and a back that angles backwards (c.110º) are health hazards. They still frequent our schools. Effectively your child is ignorantly forced to fit the mould causing him or her to sit on the base of the spine (not on the ischeal tuberosities, 'the sitting bones'). They are also rounding the back, collapsing the head back and down and the lip of the seat is cutting into the back of the thighs restricting circulation to their legs.

Leaning on the desk, twisting the body and hunching up the shoulders is all too common and all too easily becomes the harmful norm. Therefore the ideal position I have suggested when achieved is quickly experienced as uncomfortable and for some children it's "uncool".

Assuming you have invested in an adjustable chair, what can a parent do to discourage sloppy sitting? Bear with me on this. It may seem drawn out but you'll find what I am suggesting is a generational shift.

Think about how you react to sloppy sitting. I am of the generation that was told to 'sit up properly'. It did me little lasting good and caused mounting resentment. Try this. If you spot your child slouching in say a kitchen chair, ask them to be aware of their posture without immediately changing the position.

For example, "Robert I want you to remain as you are and just notice how you are sitting. Tell me how you feel".
Robert might reply, "I am twisted around and leaning on the table".
"That's what it looks like, how does it feel?"
Robert: "A bit uncomfortable."

You say, "Just think for a moment about how you can untangle yourself and get into an easier way to sit and gently let your body go there."

If you persevere with this process you have my congratulations. You are shifting your reaction to slumping (from, possibly, a repeat or your mum or dad's words) to a more interactive response that 1) gets the child to be more aware of body and posture and 2) gives the child a strategy for correcting uncomfortable posture without fuss.

A Final Word
Knowing how the body is designed to work and by utilising the Alexander Technique you become acutely aware of furniture, equipment and activities that undermine the good use of yourself.

The items mentioned above are some examples. Others would included sofas/lounge suites, the reachability of accessories, car seats, tight clothes…

Conclusions

Why do we need the Alexander Technique?
To Take Charge

Implicit in learning the Alexander Technique is a decision by you to take more responsibility for your general health and well being. If you can have more mastery of your body use and behaviours, then you lessen your dependence on others. Amongst other things, this self-reliance will cut down on the time and money you spend on health and wellness fixes elsewhere.

Basic Information and Experience:
Finding the Lost and Key Bits to the Body-Mind Jigsaw!

Were you taught how the whole body is designed and structured? How it functions? Probably not. Was time repeatedly given to how to sit well to write or compute? How much do you know about the kinesthetic sense? Possibly a little! In most cases physical education, drama, dance, and health classes in our primary and secondary education gave only sporadic information about our physical selves.

The Alexander Technique is one system that explains how the whole self operates, how it all fits together to move and position itself with ease and elegance. Most toddlers and the majority of high profile sports people have this natural essence. Most of us lose this after toddlerhood. It's just commonsense to know how our whole self should work. Armed with this self-knowledge we can prevent habits of misuse from distorting this essence.

Tertiary institutions for the performance arts have been employing Alexander Technique teachers for some time. A modified form needs to be part of the primary and secondary school curriculum. One of life's key competencies is surely being able to knowingly use yourself well.

Choosing to Change:
Responding Relatively Rationally in the Circumstances

Alexander said we 'translate everything, whether physical or mental or spiritual into muscular tension'.

By practicing the Technique in our daily round you become adept at monitoring your muscular tension. You can determine if you are unduly tense in yourself. As well, we can attend to this unnecessary state by releasing the overdoing in our muscles and find more appropriate tension for the activity.

This in itself is a handy skill to carry around. There are wider and more valuable applications for this skill. From monitoring we can see how external and internal stimuli disturb our poise.

Impulsive reactions to a command, a person, statements, circumstances, situations and events either cause us to physically open up and out in ourselves or they pull us down and in. These responses are generated by thoughts. These can be either from interpreting events external to ourselves or induced by our inner thoughts.

If we can read, hear, see or sense the barometer of muscular tension created by the stimulus, we know if it is for our good or ill. Some examples:
'Every time I drop something I bend over in a way that hurts'.
'When I think of so and so I get goose bumps and tight shoulders'.
'The sound of a siren unsettles me. I get a knot in my stomach'.
'I love to laugh it makes my body loose'.
'This child's behaviour is winding me up, I can tell because my jaw is really tight and my body feels tense'.

Alexander Technique

We react quickly to a stimulus and in most cases without really choosing our response. I am not saying we have to make conscious choices all the time (we'd never leave the house), but we can be more aware of our reactions and choose to respond differently if we consider our habitual reaction as being detrimental to our ongoing well-being.

So every time I drop something, and assuming it's not a knife through my foot, I can pause and choose any number of responses: leave the dropped item where it is, ask someone to pick it up for me or decide to follow Alexander's process of giving directions. The consequence is obvious. I have prevented the old reaction and chosen to consciously generate a new neuromuscular program. I earn myself another tick for eroding the force of the habit which previously made me bend in an injurious way.

When I catch myself thinking of so and so, I'll think to free the shoulders.
Similarly, when a siren sounds it's a cue to recall a sense of the body going up and out.
As for the kid getting on my goat: 'It's time to step outside for a while and cool off'.
Laughing is a good habit and requires no need to choose to change.

Alexander Technique as a Pleasant Background Hum in Our Lifestyle.
Once pointed out it astonishes people how much unnecessary tension resides in their bodies.

Contributing to our overall stress level are almost permanently scrunched toes, rounded shoulders, pursed lips, squinting eyes, gritted teeth, hands in a half grip shape, and tight buttocks…Discovering these tension patterns and learning how to release them constructively, is a great start in the quest to reduce stress in our lives.

Lessons with an Alexander Technique teacher will set this process in train.

The next move is finding the stimulus/stimuli that have embedded these patterns and change our response to it or them.

Controlling and eventually eliminating habits of misuse in our selves becomes an undercurrent in our thinking. My experience has been to appreciate Alexander's technique as a companion, a way to self-coach and become an ally for dealing with a world that is creating more and more stimuli.

If I didn't have a way of monitoring my response to life's demands I would be a slave of my habit that pulls my body downward and inward unknowingly. If I didn't have procedures and inner processes to assist me in maintaining good use then I'd be much less happy. If I didn't have a way of thinking that offers me a positive direction to head in, then I'd be diminished in stature and ease of movement. The Alexander Technique gives me a wide sense of integration and dignity.

These are some reasons as to why we need the Alexander Technique. For you the reader these First Steps to the Alexander Technique have possibly whet your appetite for more. I hope so. It's a very rewarding and worthwhile pursuit.

Further Reading

The Use of the Self
F.M. Alexander, (Gollancz, 1992)

The Alexander Principle
W. Barlow, (Gollancz, 1990)

Back Trouble
D. Caplan, (Compas, 1987)

Principles of the Alexander Technique
J. Chance, (Thorsons, 1998)

Body Know-How
J. Drake, (Thorsons, 1991)

The Lost Sixth Sense
D. Garlick (University of NSW, 1990)

Body Learning
M. Gelb, (Aurum Press, 1981)

The Complete Illustrated Guide to the Alexander Technique
G. Macdonald (Element Book, 1998)

The Art of Changing
G Park,(Ashgrove Press, 1989)

Useful Addresses

Chris Raff (Author)
PO Box 1202,
Aldinga Beach, SA 5173.
Tel: 08 85565651.

Australian Society of Teachers of the Alexander Technique
(AUSTAT) Inc.
PO Box 716
Darlinghurst NSW 2010
Tel: 1800 339 571
www.alexandertechnique.org.au

The Society provides a list of qualified teachers throughout
Australia.

*This directory is full of helpful information and overseas
addresses.*

The Journey of a Thousand Miles Begins with a First Step...

First Steps
series

- First Steps to Meditation
- First Steps to Massage
- First Steps to Chi Kung
- First Steps to Tarot
- First Steps to Dream Power
- First Steps to Yoga
- First Steps to Palmistry
- First Steps to Feng Shui
- First Steps to Managing Stress
- First Steps to Astrology
- First Steps to Acupressure
- First Steps to Alexander Technique
- First Steps to Numerology

Further titles following shortly